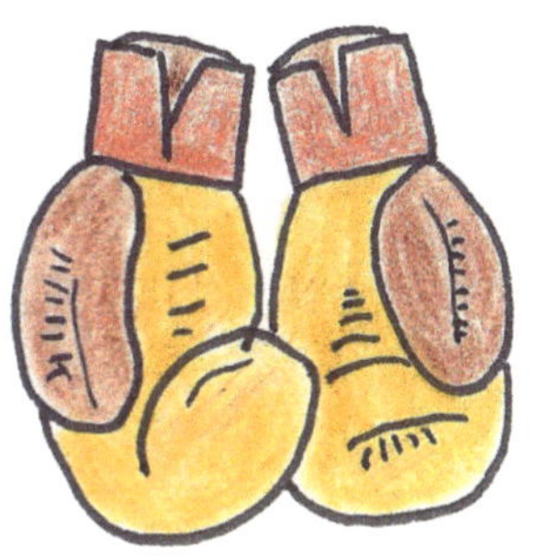

STEADY AS A ROCK

WRITTEN & ILLUSTRATED BY

ANNA COHN DONNELLY

*I lovingly dedicate this book to the real boxer in the family—
CJD who is firmly by my side on this unexpected journey.*

PREFACE

This is the story about a unique group of mostly senior citizens who are turned into 'fighters' by their boxing coach Nelson. What are they fighting? Parkinson's Disease. Nelson gives them hope for a better future. It's the first time in many years that many of them have felt hope, not shame and despair. It's the first time they don't hide their shaking hands. I know. I am a member of the group.

Our opponent is a degenerative progressive brain disease, but we all believe that we will defeat this foe. We will train and we will box. This disease will not win. Even though we might look old and shaky, we've discovered that we are all fighters. And that is what the class Nelson teaches, called Rock Steady Boxing, is all about—replacing despair with hope—the belief that we are not alone and as a group we are stronger and can run, squat, box, and move in ways we never thought possible.

We work out hard. And, we have fun. Sometimes we work out to our favorite music—music from the 60's and 70's—and for a brief time we don't feel like Parkinson's patients at all. Rather, we feel like the young carefree adults we once were before Parkinson's controlled our movement.

To a casual observer we may limp and shake and look frail. We know that each day is a battle and we refuse to surrender—no matter how unrelenting our foe is. We are now fighters…1 2 3 ROCK STEADY!

Judy M.
PD Patient and Boxer

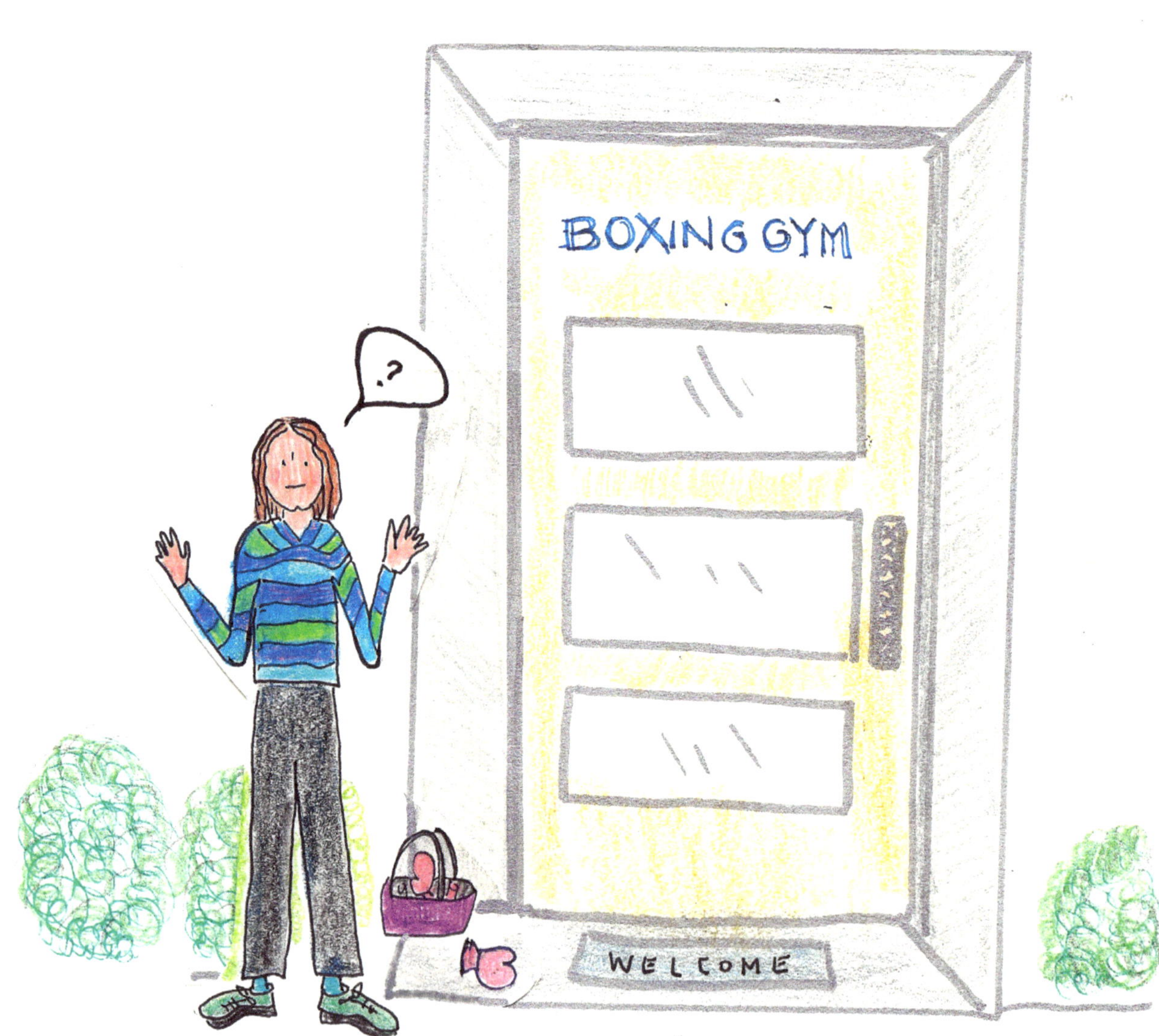

?
BOXING GYM
WELCOME

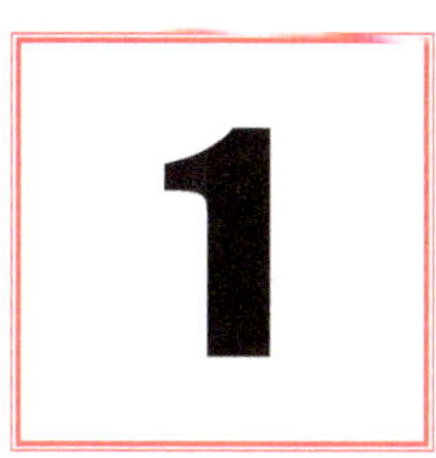

1

WHAT AM I DOING HERE?

I think of myself as a gentle person. How did I end up at a boxing gym? I'd never been drawn to boxing.

Let's go back in time a bit. It was the 10th of November 2015. I got an email from my brother David titled "Rock Steady Boxing." He wrote:

> *Anna: Have you heard of a program called "Rock Steady Boxing"? It teaches Parkinson's patients how to box, and the results, as reported on CBS Sunday Morning this week, are very good. Call me and I'll explain. David*

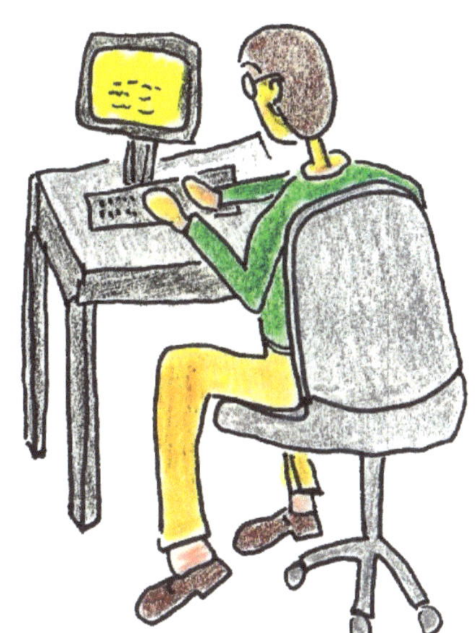

Five years earlier, I had been handed the shocking diagnosis of Parkinson's, or "PD." I knew nothing about the disease. I knew no one who had it. I learned all too soon that it is a neurological, progressive, degenerative disease with no known cure. The news was devastating at first. It took a number of months to realize that PD was not a death sentence but rather something I had to accommodate myself to and to manage.

My doctor, a neurologist and movement disorder specialist, prescribed medication, vigorous exercise, a healthy diet, and reduced stress.

So I set about doing some exercise most every day - alternating biking and yoga, and doing weights with a trainer, and walking on a treadmill. I watched what I ate. I pulled back from some of my work. I took several different PD medications.

In time, my symptoms—tremor, poor handwriting, quiet voice, stiffness, clumsiness, curled toes, low blood pressure—were somewhat controlled. But, I was far from being in great shape. I was pretty self-conscious about having PD. And, while I had major support from my family and friends, and had great doctors, I was mostly managing it on my own.

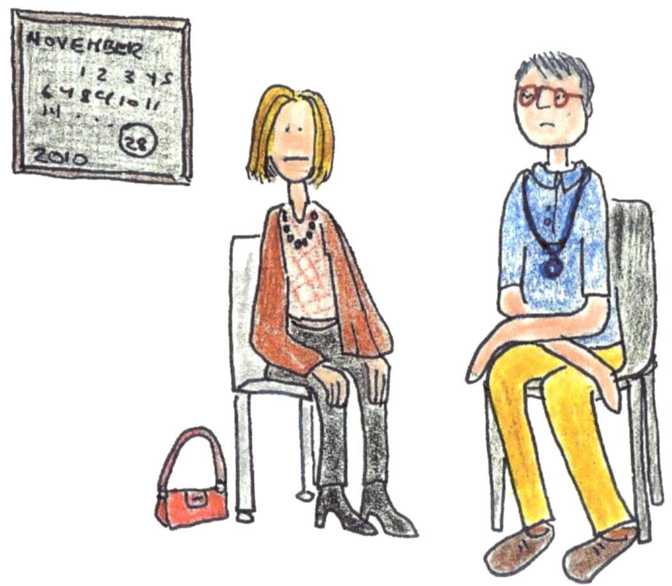

I called David. He explained what he saw on the CBS segment with Leslie Stahl and urged me to watch the piece, and then find a Rock Steady Boxing program near me, and enroll. Boxing? Really? But David was adamant and then my sister-in-law Naida got on the phone and said, "*You HAVE to do it!*" And so I did. After all, when Naida said "do it", you "did it".

I watched the segment. Looked interesting! Near me? Fat chance! I checked out Rock Steady Boxing online at their website at www.rocksteadyboxing.org. I was surprised to learn that the class was offered at a boxing gym twenty minutes from my home, and right near our mom, Mimi. Even though I still couldn't see myself boxing, I wrote back:

> *David and Naida: Check this out. There is a boxing gym 20 minutes away that offers Rock Steady Boxing classes. I think I'll go explore it with a visit. Love you.*

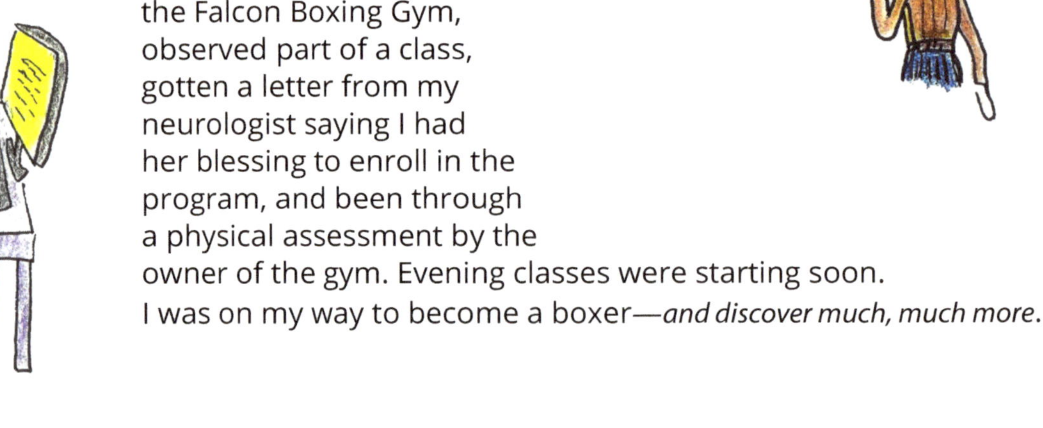

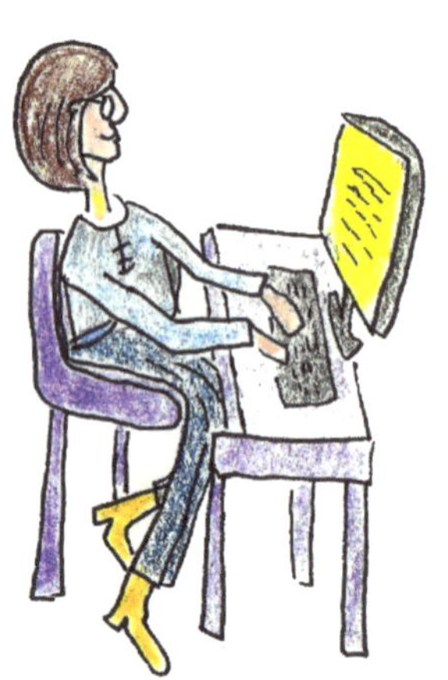

Within a week I had toured the Falcon Boxing Gym, observed part of a class, gotten a letter from my neurologist saying I had her blessing to enroll in the program, and been through a physical assessment by the owner of the gym. Evening classes were starting soon. I was on my way to become a boxer—*and discover much, much more*.

2

FALCON BOXING GYM TOUR

I found The Falcon Boxing Gym to be an amazing place. It was new and spacious and filled with state of the art boxing equipment and then some.

Floor Plan of Gym

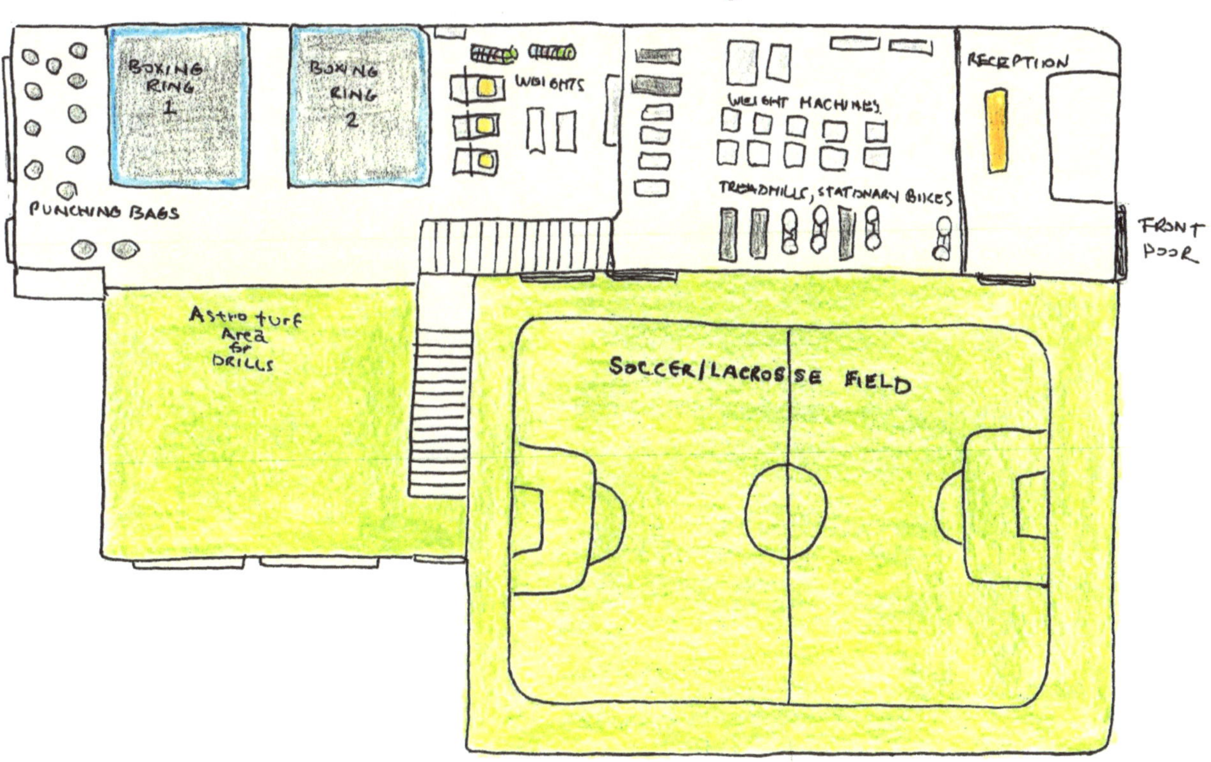

It included:

- a regulation size indoor Astroturf soccer field that was also used for lacrosse,
- two boxing rings,
- several dozen punching bags of various sizes and shapes,
- a few speed bags,
- a comprehensive collection of strength training equipment,
- five treadmills,
- several stationary bikes,
- a few elliptical machines,
- weights of all sizes and poundage,
- a large turf covered area for drills,
- ropes,
- truck tires and more.

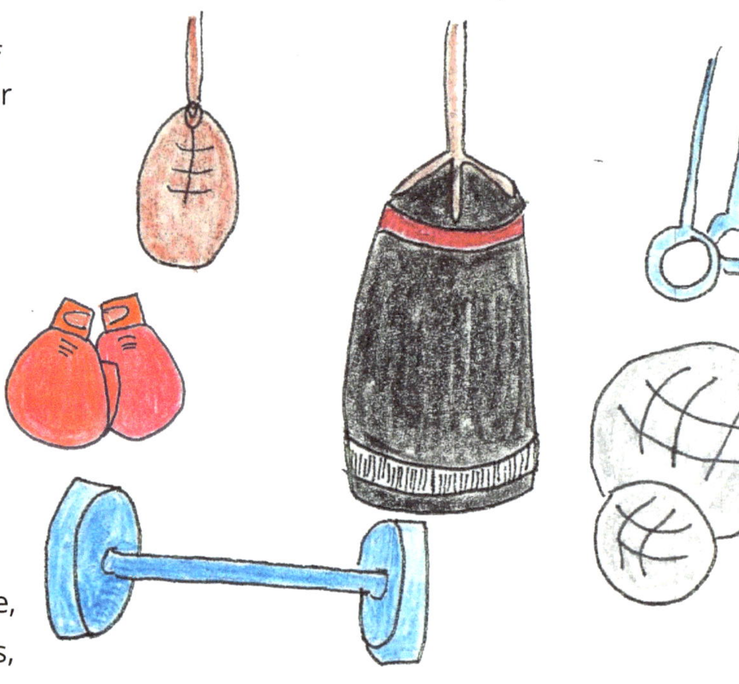

The gym's soccer field was heavily used by local sports clubs—some school age, some more senior. Several personal trainers worked one-on-one with clients in the boxing area and also taught boxing classes. And then there were the Rock Steady Boxing folks. They were surrounded by athletes of all ages and types. They didn't really stand out—just one more group working on the equipment and the bags.

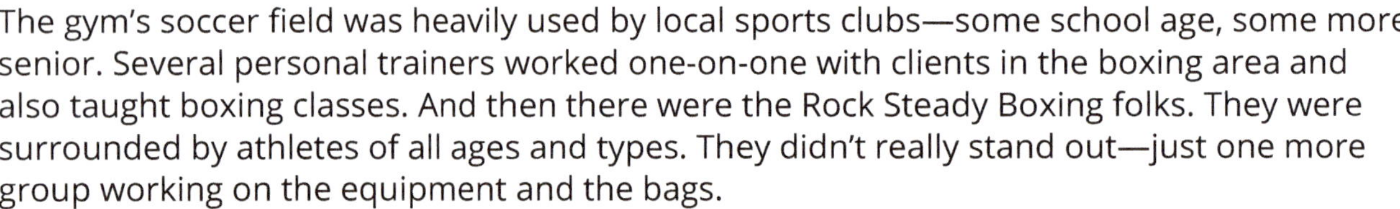

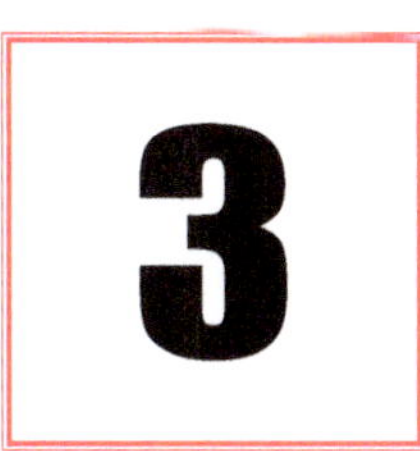

THE FIRST CLASS

The first Monday in December I showed up for my first class. Even though I had toured the gym a few weeks earlier and watched part of a class, I stood by my car in the parking lot for a bit, anxious about going in. I hadn't really spent too much time around people with PD and I didn't know what it might be like working out with some of them. I wasn't sure what to expect. But I had promised David and Naida I would try it out and so I willed myself to go on in.

I don't remember exactly how many people were there—maybe eight or nine. In time our numbers grew.

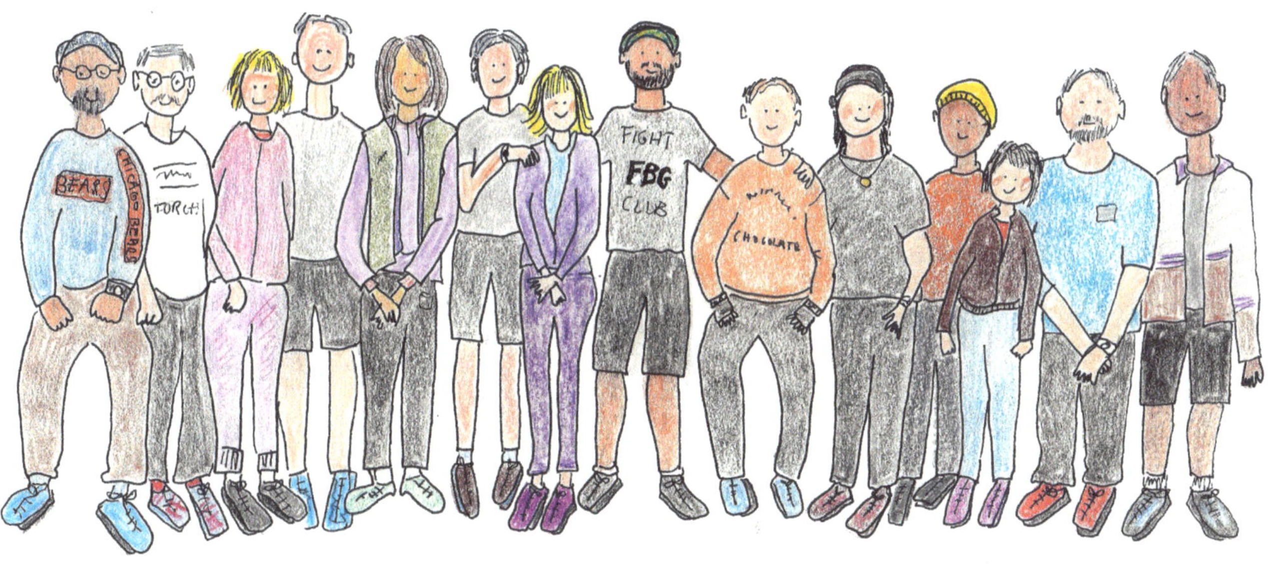

I also don't remember if or how we were introduced to each other. We didn't talk to each other very much. A few seemed to know each other. I later learned that some were couples—one spouse supporting the other. Most of my attention was focused on Nelson, our trainer, and trying to do what he was asking us to do. And trying to not have my PD tremor show.

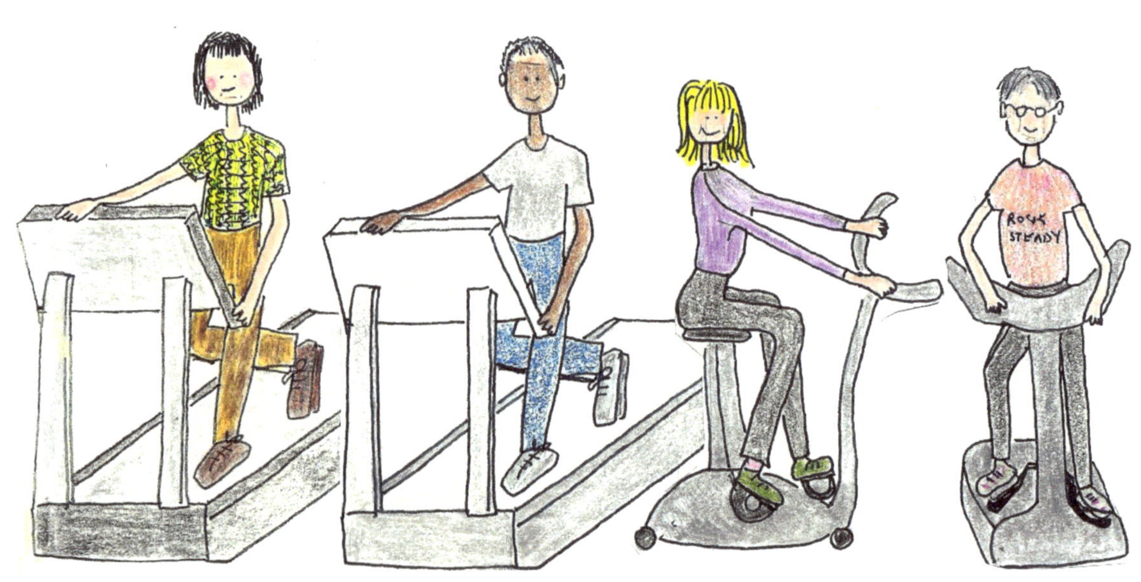

ROCK
STEADY

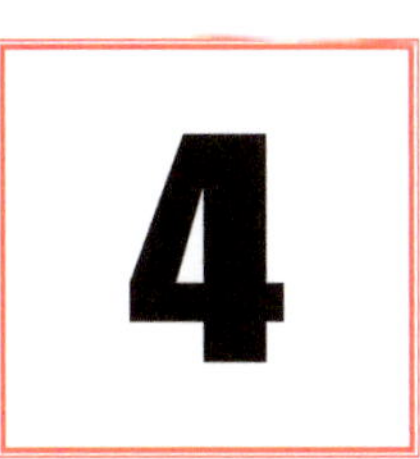

THE ROCK STEADY BOXING ROUTINE

I survived my first class and started to go on a regular basis. Soon enough I came to understand the Rock Steady Boxing routine and just what challenges it presented to me.

The class lasted one and one-half hours and was offered six times a week—three at night and three in the afternoon. Our trainer Nelson recommended we come at least three times a week. And that is what I have tried to do. Of course, life has a way of interfering with the best laid plans.

I found it to be a very difficult routine. Spouses or other family members were welcome to participate in classes. Several did regularly. Members of my family—Chris, Kaitlin, Kathe, David, Amy, Julie, and Becky have all come with me. They all agreed. It is a tough workout whether you have PD or not.

We start on bikes or the treadmill or the elliptical and get a good 10 to 15 minutes of aerobic warm up. I was on familiar territory here. Then, onto 15 minutes of stretching—one intense yoga class in a quarter of an hour—*my cup of tea!*

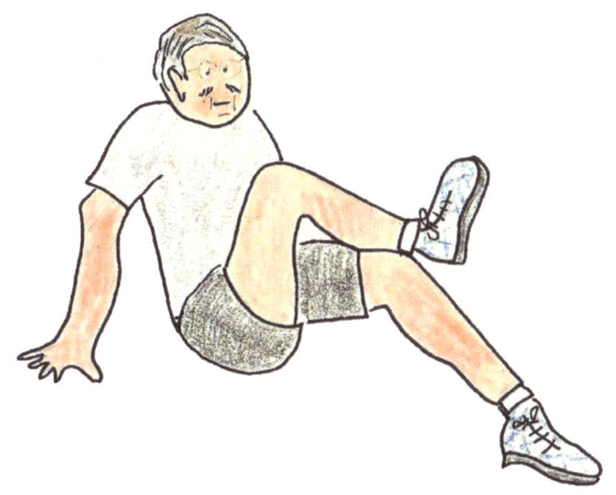

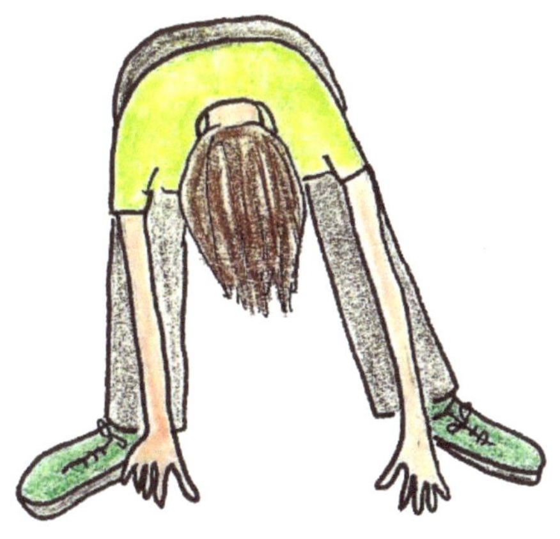

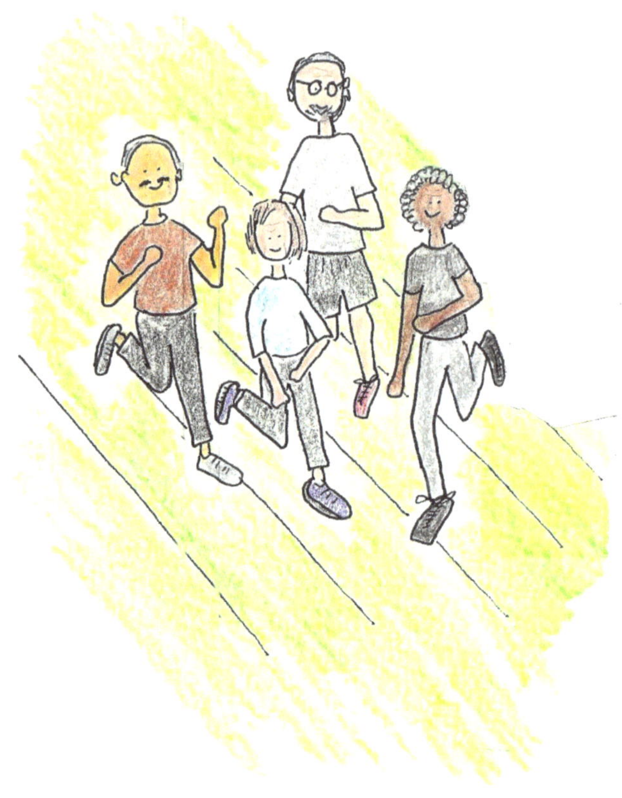

Next we do a variety of drills. If the soccer/lacrosse field is open we might do a series of jogs; then sprints across the field and back; some high knees and butt kick laps, and some running backwards interspersed with jumping jacks, push-ups, and squats. I am usually huffing and puffing by now.

With only a few moments to get a sip of water and catch my breath, we are onto a variety of exercises in a circuit with weights, tires, stairs, ropes— an intense TRX-type program in 20 minutes—lots of strength work plus work on balance. None are easy for me.

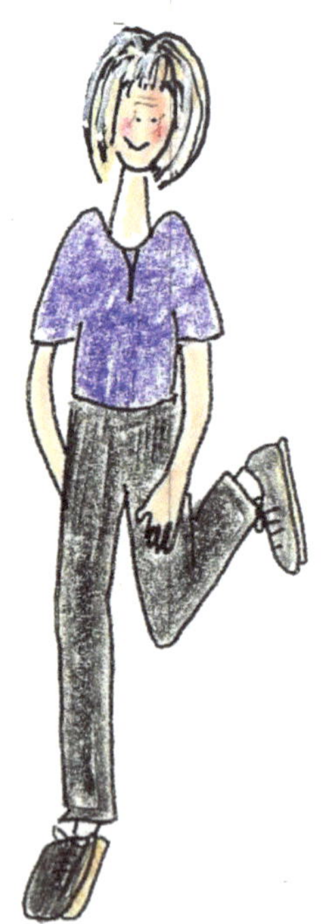

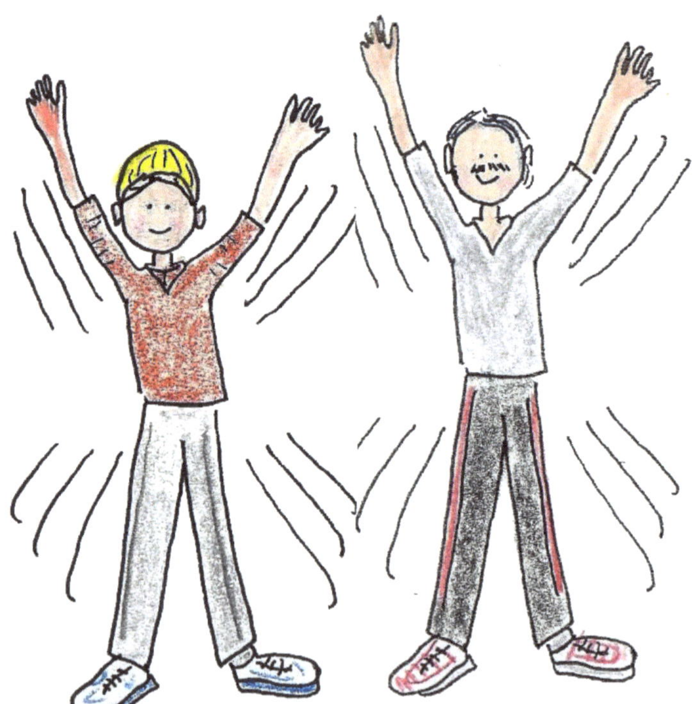

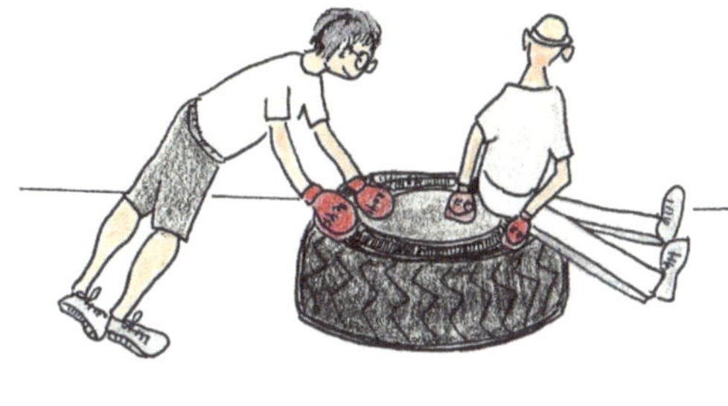

THE TIRE DRILL: One drill is to lean on a giant tire and alternate push-ups with sideways steps around the tire. After one loop you turn around and go the other way. No big deal at first. After several loops though my arms always turn to noodles, my breath is out of control, and I am tripping over my feet—coordination matters here.

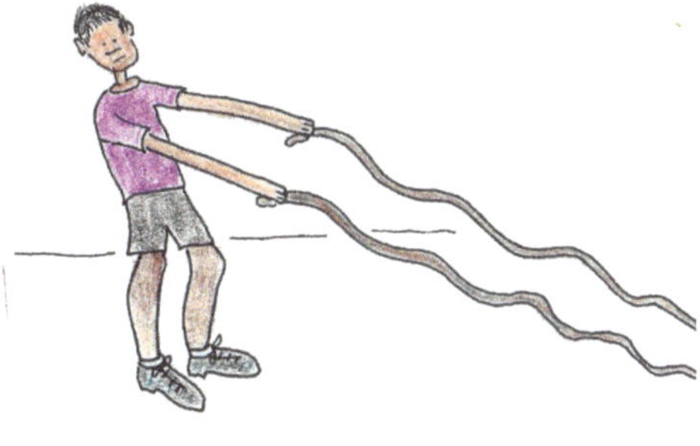

THE BATTLE ROPES: I hate the ropes. We work with two ropes. It seems they each weigh a hundred pounds and the idea is to hold one in each hand, squat, and wave them up and slam them down quickly creating ripples going down the rope. This uses every muscle in my core and then some. When I do the ropes, my stomach aches...my arms ache...my back aches. And it doesn't seem to ever get any easier. The ropes are "Pilates-Plus."

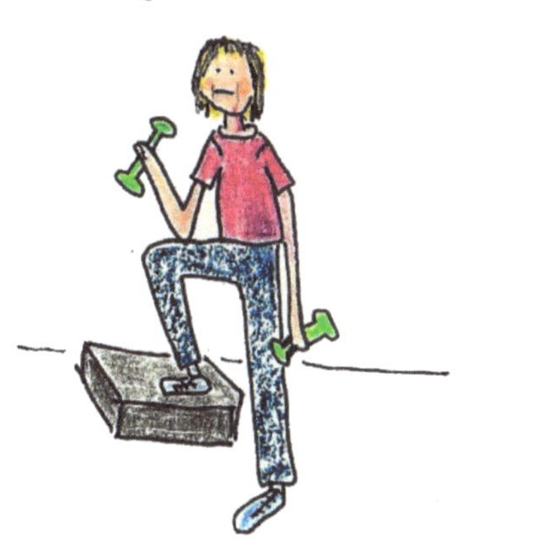

THE STEP-UP DRILL: Another drill that seems so easy really isn't for me. Nelson says, "Holding weights in each hand, simply step up on this block and lift one weight and then the other in the air. Step down. Then switch legs." Simple, right? Wait until you've done it 10 times. My arms begin to rebel. My legs do too. And soon enough I am only stepping up on the left leg and only raising the right arm. This is more than a physical exercise. It is mental as well. And it's about balance.

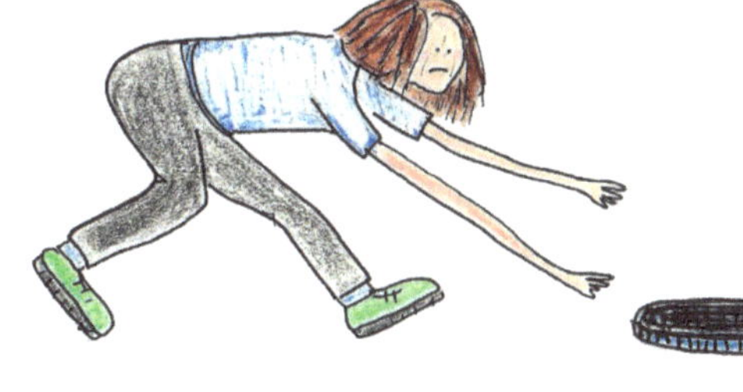

THE BEAR CRAWL: Then there are the dreaded bear crawls. All we are asked to do is crawl forward for 20 feet on our hands and feet—not our hands and knees—pushing a 25 pound weight, and then crawl backwards for 20 feet, pulling the weight. Maybe babies and bears can do this easily. It requires coordination and endurance. *My whole body aches!*

We may finish off our drills with running up and down the stairs two at a time.

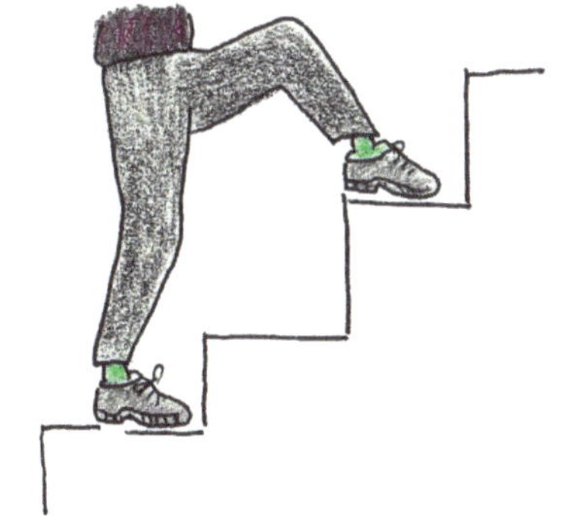

Totally out of breath, we turn to boxing—putting on our wraps and boxing gloves. Mine are pink, bubble gum pink. We prepare to punch a very heavy bag or spar in the ring with our trainer.

First we assume the boxer's stance. With my hands held high protecting my face, I stand sideways to the punching bag with knees slightly bent and my back leg supporting my balance—this isn't a natural pose to me. Hitting the bag hard isn't natural either. Nelson tells us to throw our punches with more than our hands, but twist our entire body into the punch. I try.

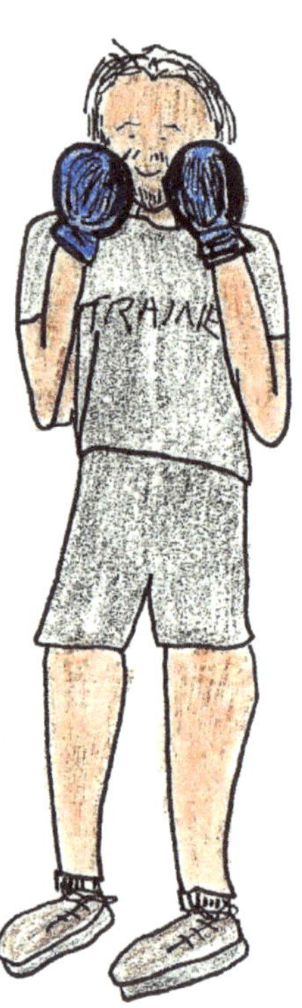

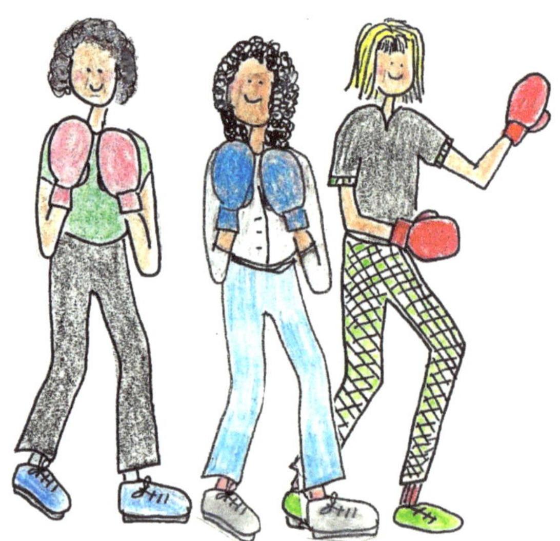

Nelson has us box at two minute intervals, with 30 second breaks after each, for 20 minutes or so. At first, moving my feet while punching was impossible. I felt like a marble statue, fixed in place, but with arms that moved—awkwardly. Slowly I learned to shuffle my feet a bit as I punched, then to hop, and finally to move with a bit of a rhythm.

Next I had to conquer my stamina deficiency. Punching fast or slow after several two-minute intervals was hard at first. And it still is. But I do move more and punch harder.

It's a good workout!

Nelson borrowed a diagram originally created for Mike Tyson to use for us "PD" boxers, assigning numbers seemingly randomly to different punches and jabs directed at various parts of the body. He yells out number sequences, often coupled with an exercise for us to follow. He came up with this so we are challenging both sides of our brains even as we work out.

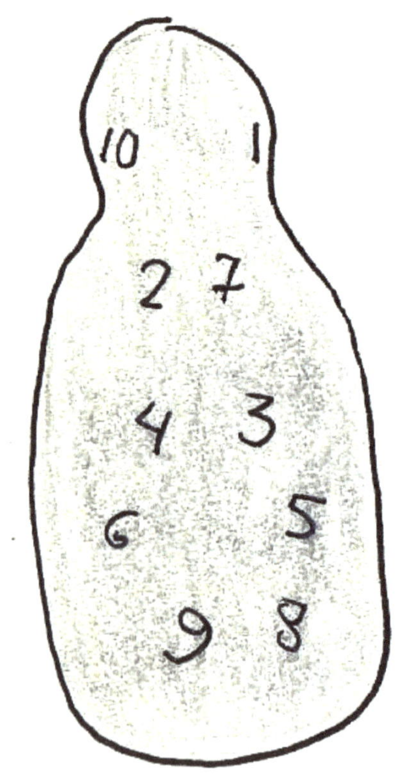

"7-7-2-7-2-7-2-5-9-9-2!"

Rapid fire "3-4's." "Take the squat." Rapid fire "5-9's."

High knees and "7-2's."

Inevitably jumping jacks, hard in any case, but torture with boxing gloves on.

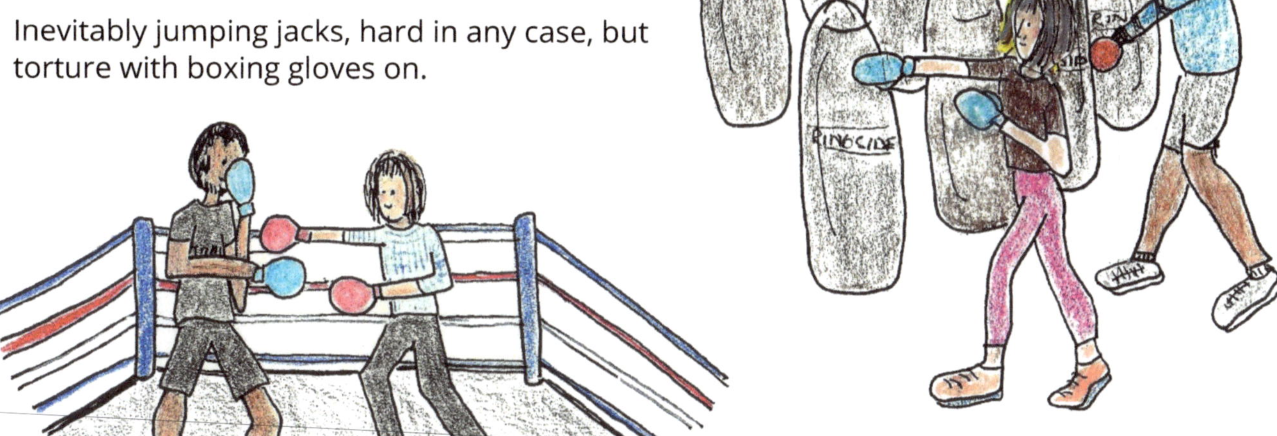

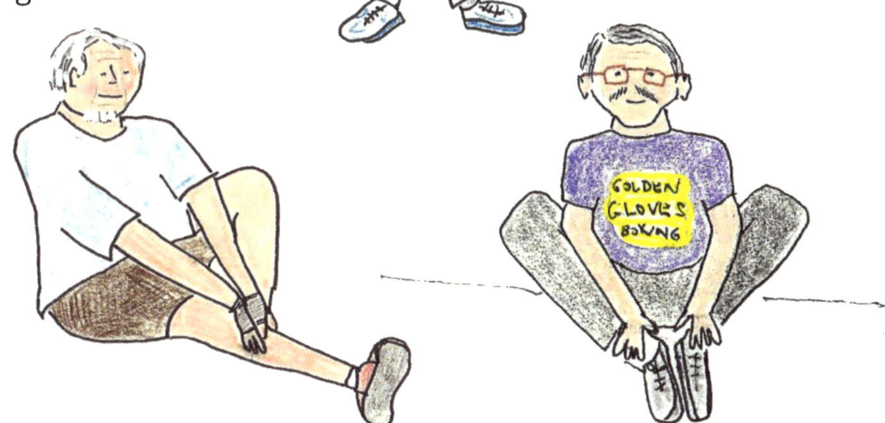

It has taken me months to get all the numbers and punches straight. And, I am still not sure I have them right. This "PD" boxing is more than physical work—it is definitely brain work as well.

Finally, we return to stretching.

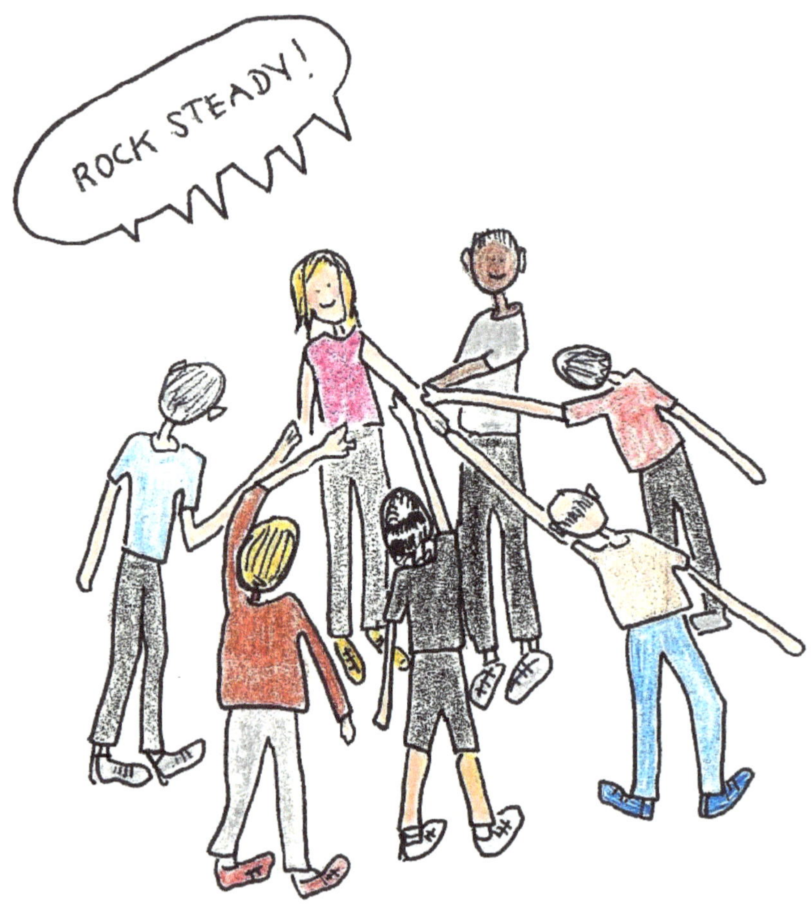

To close out the class we stand in a huddle, we each put one hand in the middle and—after the count of one, two, three—yell "**ROCK STEADY!**"

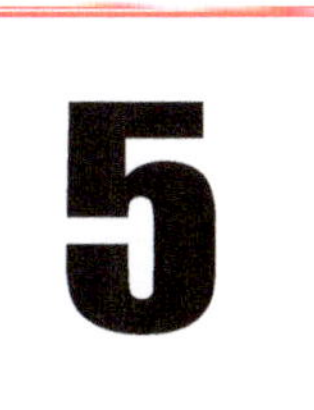

5

BUDDING FRIENDSHIPS

I was very self-conscious in class at first. The tremor in my left hand would start up as I began to stretch and would come back while boxing. I couldn't control it. But then, I noticed that others with PD had the identical tremor. And, some people were bent over or dragged one foot or were stiff, very stiff. And none of us were nimble or quick. There was really no reason to be self-conscious in this group.

Ever so slowly conversations among my classmates began. Initially most of the banter was about typical casual topics:

"How about those Cubs!"

"Where do you drive from to get here?"

"Can you believe all the rain we are getting?"

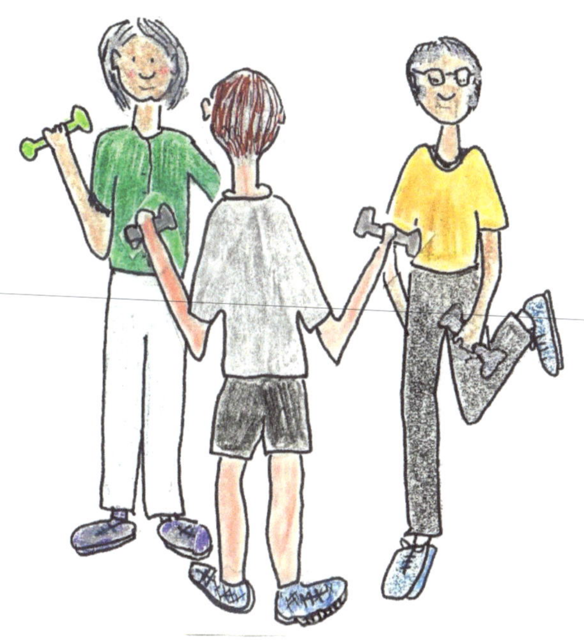

The talk slowly turned to PD.

"How did you discover Rock Steady Boxing?"

"When were you diagnosed?"

"Who is your doctor?"

As time went by, inevitably our conversations about PD broadened—as did our conversations about life.

"There is a PD support group meeting at Glenbrook hospital next Thursday if you are interested."

"I just heard about a new medical device for PD."

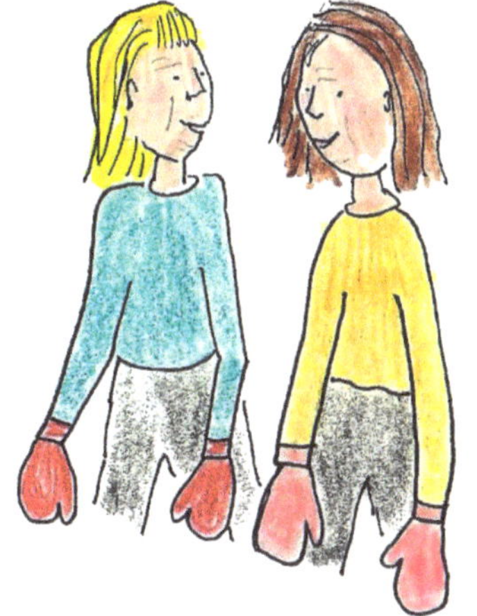

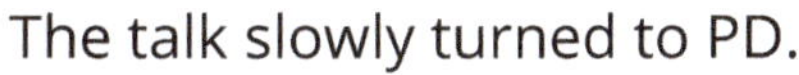

Soon enough my classmates and I were sharing the more personal and sensitive challenges of PD.

"What were your symptoms when you were diagnosed?" "Oh, my daughter said I was tripping all the time and I noticed I was dragging my foot. And you?"

"With PD my toes curl. Do yours?" "I have the same thing! I found some toe straighteners on-line. I'll give you one to try out."

"Are you stiff all the time? I am." "I was but I now use the PD patch and love it. Last summer I went to a wedding and simply couldn't dance. I didn't realize how stiff I was. I got out on the dance floor and couldn't move around. Weeks later I started using the patch. And now I can dance to my heart's content … tap, cha-cha– well, sort of. I can even do jumping jacks.–well, sort of."

"What pills do you take?"

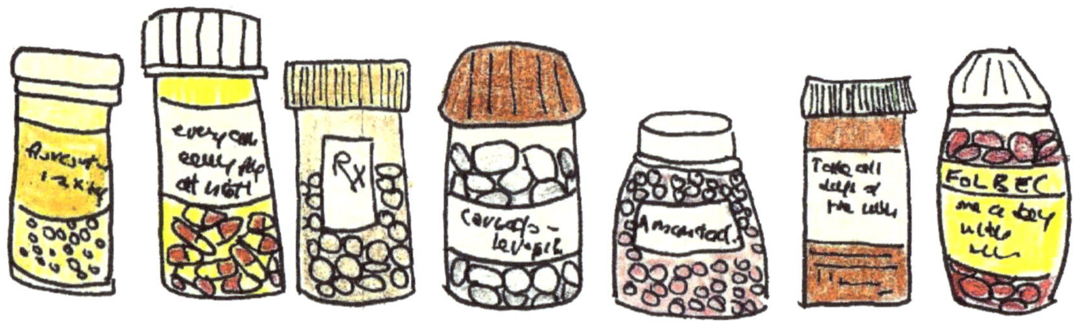

A rude question in most any social situation but not for us. It is part of our typical conversations. It seem that everyone was taking different medications. And everyone had tried things that didn't work. A common response might be:

"I tried that and couldn't sleep."

"I used it for five days and broke out in hives."

"It didn't do anything for me."

Or,

"Tell me more—maybe I'll discuss it with my doctor."

And some of what my boxing mates shared was hard to listen to:

"The pain from my PD is intolerable some days. My legs cramp and I can barely get out of bed in the morning, but my doctor may be giving me a prescription for strong pain killers."

"I am totally depressed most of the time from PD. I take pills for it but they don't help. Even coming here doesn't seem to help that much. But it is better than doing nothing!"

"With PD at times it is hard to see a bright future."

Sometimes I learned something about a drug I'd never heard of. And about combinations of drugs people use. Sometimes I reported on new drugs or research I had heard of. Most of us seemed resigned to the fact that trial and error with drugs is and will be a constant in our lives … and that the pill to stop PD doesn't exist yet; but we are all convinced that without Rock Steady Boxing things would be worse.

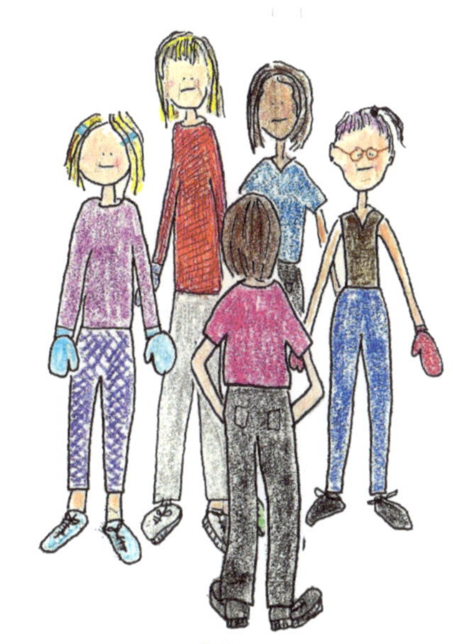

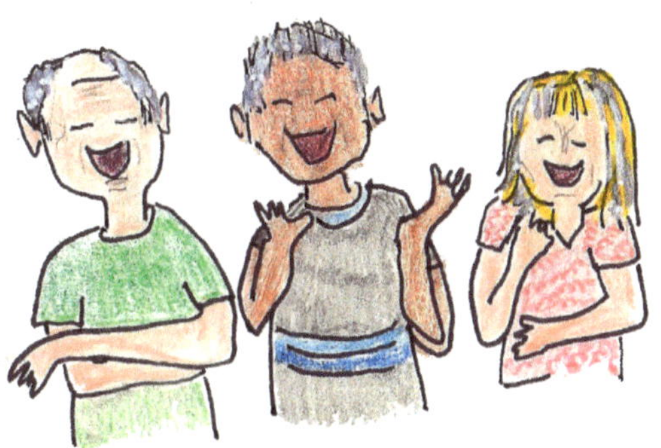

Not long after we began to share our PD stories, the teasing and joking around started, first between Nelson and a couple of the guys. And then between Nelson and all of us. And then, amongst the group at large, from time-to-time, laughter rang throughout the gym.

And, we had fun.

Dancing to the background music or singing to oldies but goodies as we boxed.

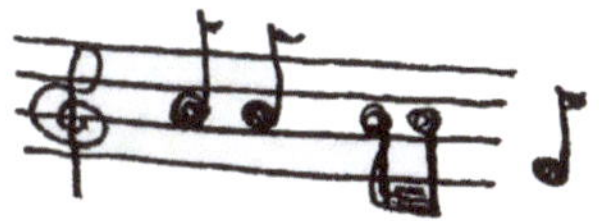

Nelson always pushed us. The workouts were hard. They never got any easier. Not after one month or three or six or twelve, for that matter.

"Come on Anna, you can go faster than that!"

"Roman, add more weight, you can do it!"

"George, get down in that squat or everyone will do 20 push-ups!"

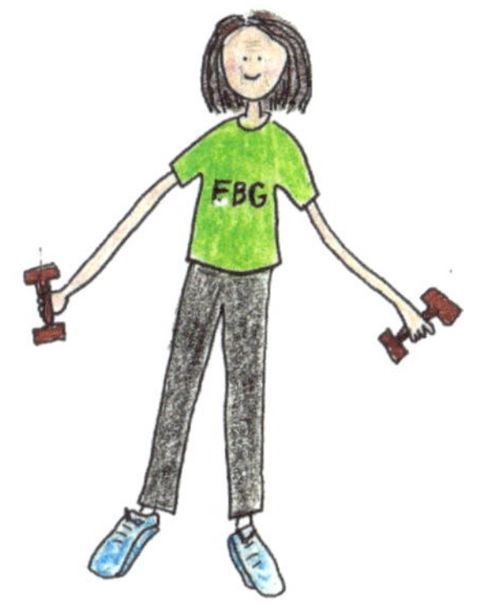

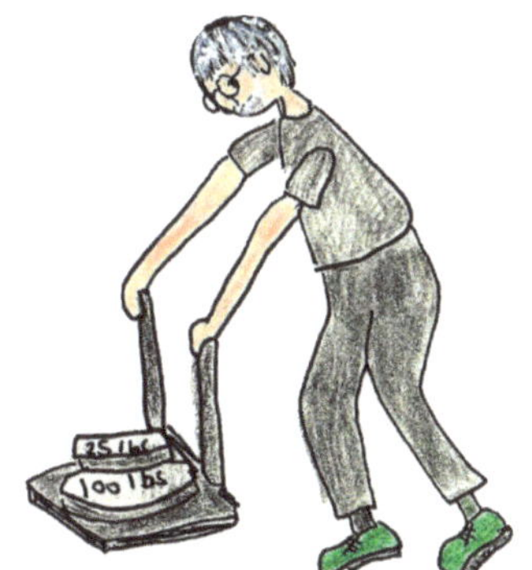

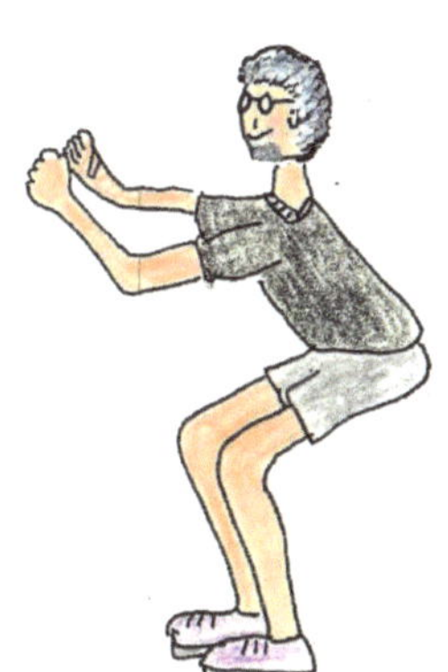

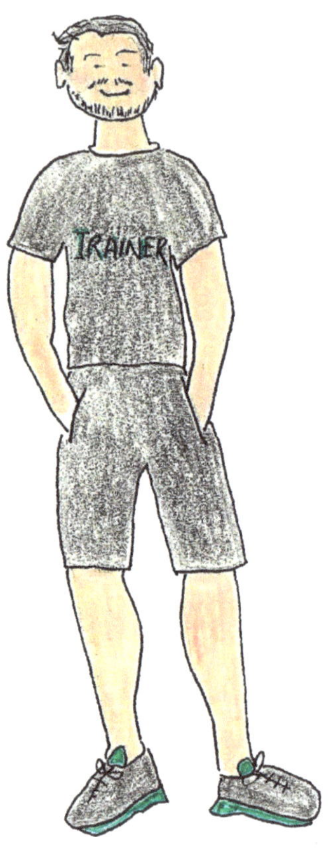

Nelson never pushed too hard. He seemed to have a sense of when I or others were on the verge of not being OK and he pulled back.

> *"Pat, why not get some water."*

> *"That's fine Judy, you can slow down."*

> *"Chuck, sit down for a minute."*

Even as we were being pushed, something interesting was happening. Perhaps we were getting stronger. Perhaps not. Perhaps the progression of our PD was slowing. Perhaps not. But we were certainly getting more comfortable with each other and we were getting closer.

An unlikely group of people. People who under any other circumstance might never have crossed paths. And, here we were cheering each other on:

> *"You can do it John!"*

> *"Go Dennis go!"*

> *"Way to go Dan!"*

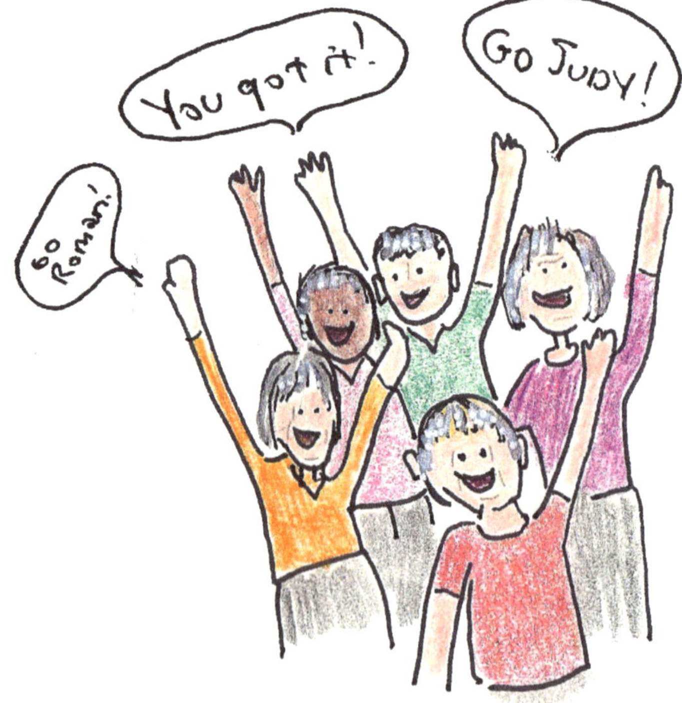

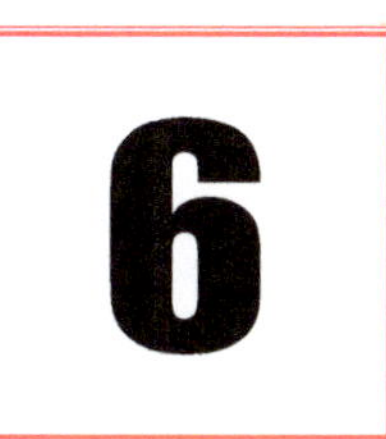

THE FALCON GYM FAMILY

Over the course of eighteen months, several dozen people came to our evening class. Some came once or twice. Some came for a number of months and dropped out for a while or altogether. Everyone new was welcomed and everyone who had been gone for a while and came back was greeted with great enthusiasm.

For most of the eighteen months, the same small group of people was regularly at class.

At the start of class I always did my aerobic warm up on the same treadmill … ten minutes uphill at a good pace. Almost always John and Roman were on the stationary bikes right next to "my" treadmill when I arrived. Their bikes were situated right in front of a window looking out on the soccer field. We'd gab back and forth about news of the day and then some.

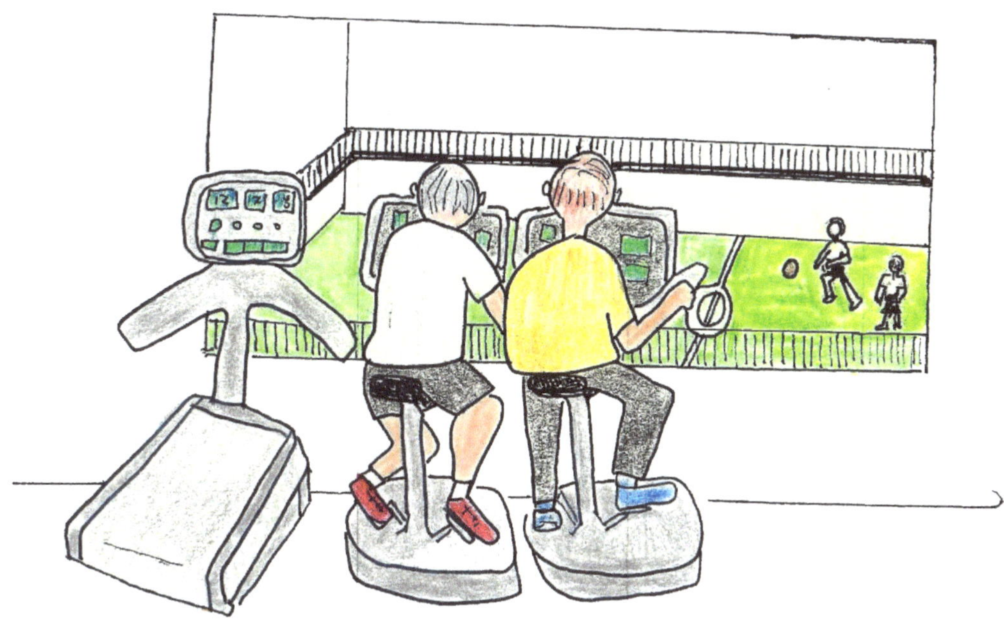

Often, shortly thereafter, Dennis would show up and hop on a bike. Then Judy and her husband Dan—she on the elliptical and he on the treadmill. And then Pat and her husband Chuck—both on treadmills. And George would show up a few moments late and just yak with everyone. Others might also show up but that was our core group. We noticed if someone didn't show up. We delighted when everyone did. We clearly cared about each other.

> When Pat had surgery and had to sit out of class for a month and gear up slowly upon her return, we were concerned.

> When George couldn't get his blood pressure under control and had to skip class, we worried.

> And when Judy discovered she had a hair line fracture on her leg, and had to wear a boot for six weeks, we sympathized.

Simply put: *we were there for each other.*

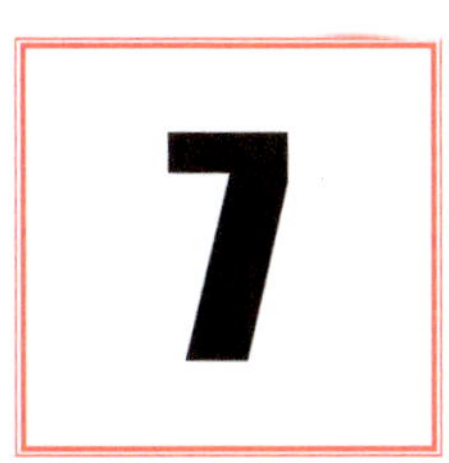

7

AND SO…

Winter turned into spring, spring to summer, then fall and winter again, and then spring. Most of us had been working out together for almost 18 months. As our workouts continued so did our conversations.

We were members of an exclusive club—**The PD Club**—a club no one would ask to join. Our guards were lowered with each other; we trusted each other. We could discuss most anything with each other without being judged. We were indeed friends.

For me, no matter what had happened in my world on any given day, no matter how stressed or tired or down I felt, once our core group assembled and we were warming up, I could count on two things for sure:

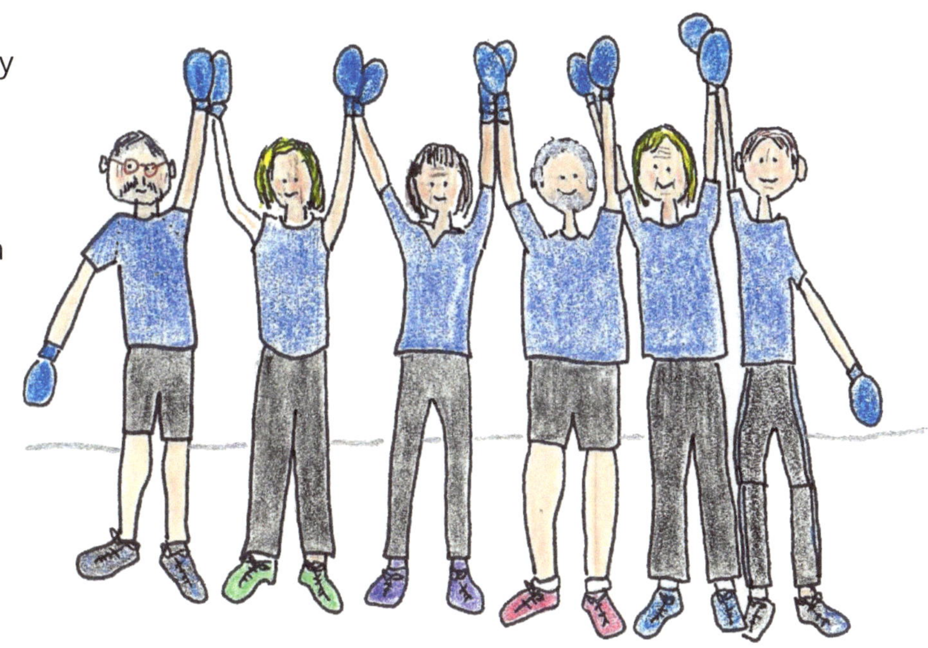

> One, I knew I would feel better at the end of class, physically and emotionally.

> And two, I knew I would be surrounded by understanding friends doing something very challenging but also enjoyable.

No one of us would be fighting PD by ourselves.

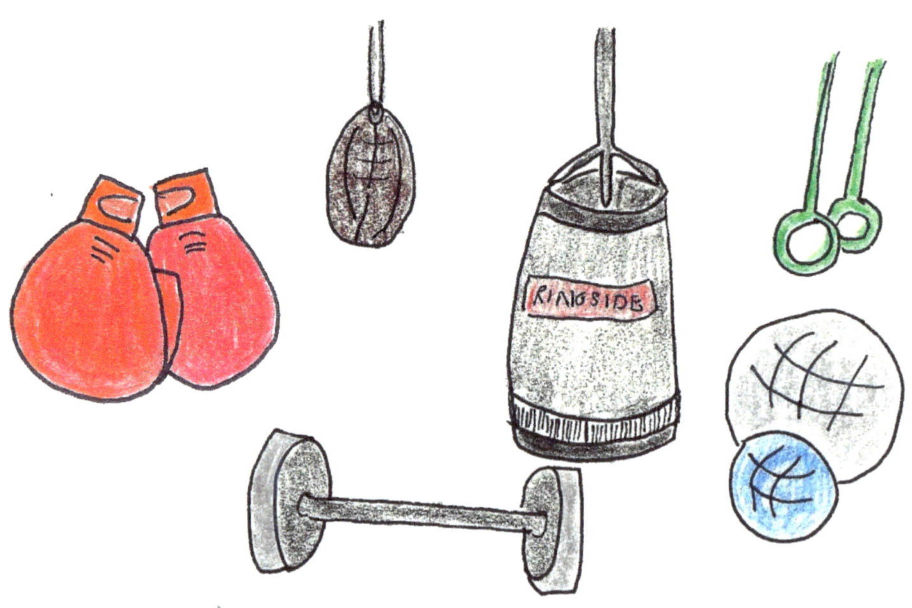

RINGSIDE

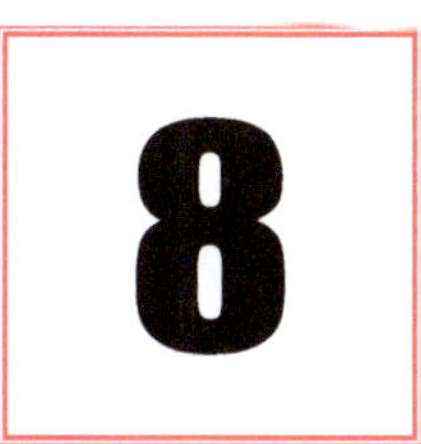# ROLL WITH THE PUNCHES

I developed a beautiful routine. I would drive the fifteen minutes from my house to Mimi's (my mom) at The Glen an hour before class. I would visit with her for half an hour, catch up, and sip a cup of tea, then drive the five additional minutes to the Falcon Boxing Gym. Mimi had just turned 97. These visits were precious.

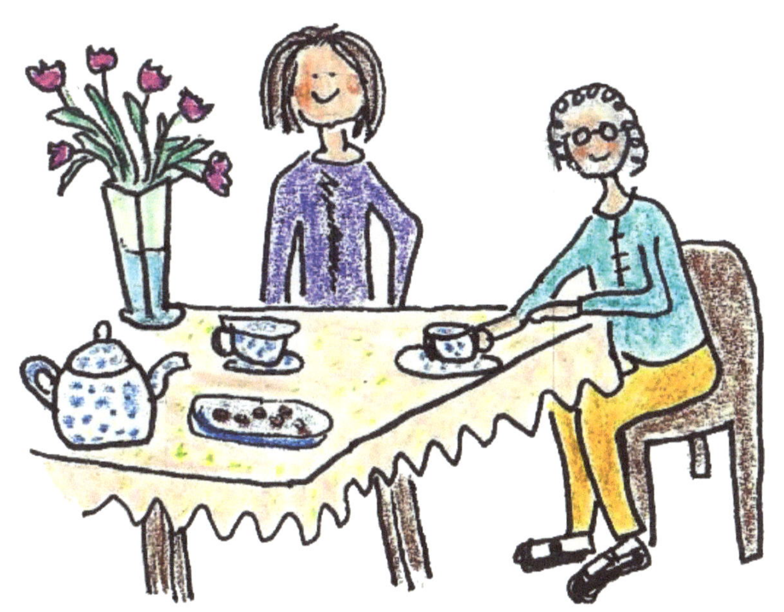

We had each developed a routine around attending our boxing classes. That was about to end.

One day Nelson announced: "Starting June 1st, classes will be at the Rumi Maki Gym in Palatine. And, we may meet at different times."

He had told us months earlier, that in the late spring we would probably have to leave the Falcon Boxing Gym. Nelson explained that the owners planned to convert the gym into an indoor soccer training center. There would be no way to accommodate Rock Steady or any boxing for that matter. At the time, late spring was months away. And, I guess I never believed it would happen. I think most of us didn't believe it. Each of us had grown to love the Falcon Boxing Gym and all we did there.

But Palatine it was to be.

Palatine? That was at least fortyfive minutes away from where I live, and probably a lot longer during rush hour. And, Mimi was not on the way. I felt like I had been punched in the stomach. It would be a change and a much longer commute for most of us.

The question was *"Could I roll with the punch?"* I needed to determine how important Rock Steady Boxing with Nelson—our trainer—and this group of people was to me. We each did.

Turned out it was not a hard decision afterall.

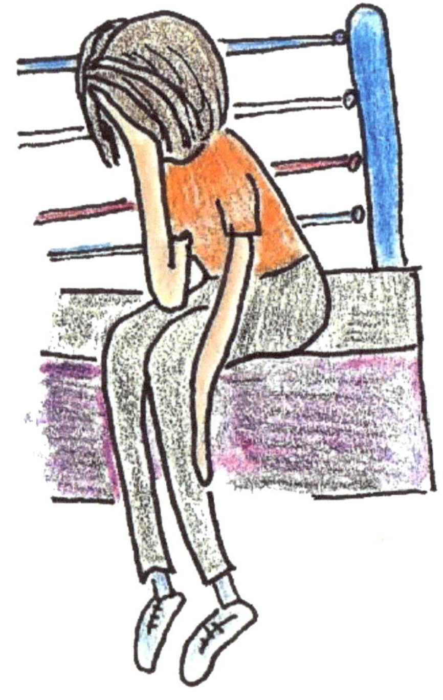

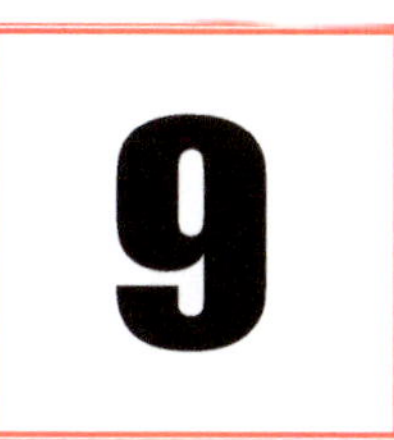

GOING THE DISTANCE

The last day together at the Falcon Boxing Gym arrived. At the end of class we gathered in a huddle and each put an arm in and we all counted "one, two, three" and yelled "ROCK STEADY!" just as we had done eighteen months ago, at my first class. It felt different now. We were a team in a huddle, getting pumped for a big fight. And in a way I guess we were.

It is the fight against PD. It feels good. It's nice to be part of a team. Nice to be a part of this team.

I THINK WE ARE ALL LOOKING FORWARD TO BEING TOGETHER NEXT WEEK IN OUR NEW GYM.

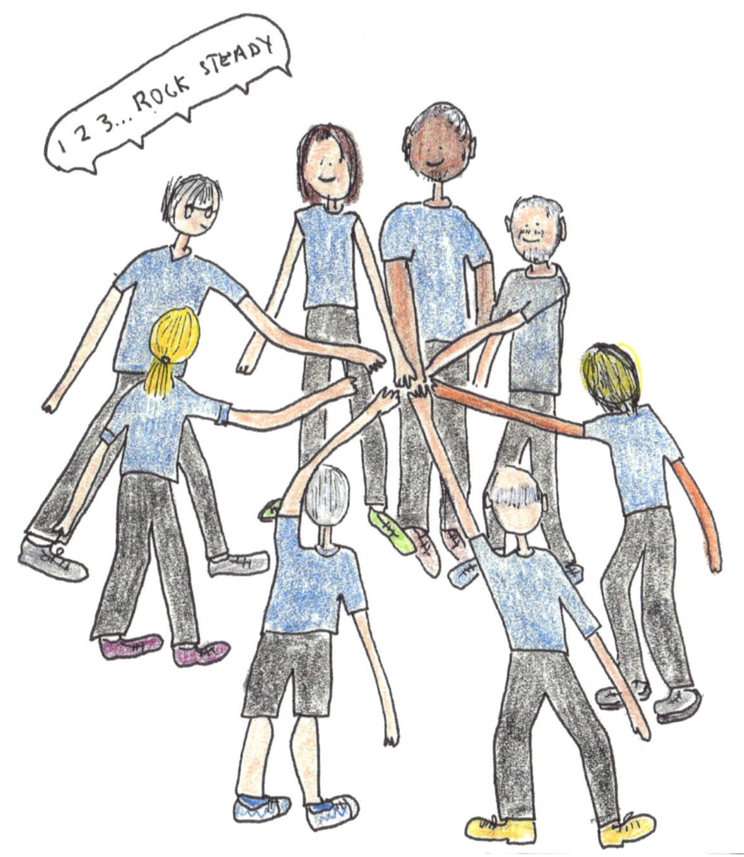

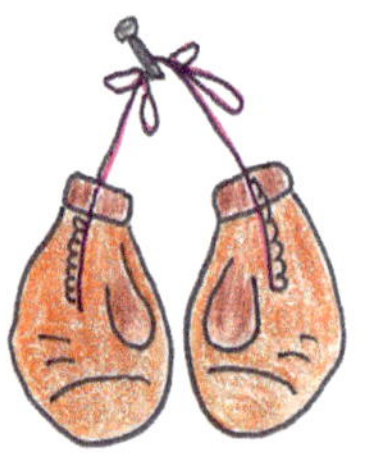

For more information about Rock Steady Boxing
and fighting back against Parkinson's, visit:
www.rocksteadyboxing.org

Books by author & illustrator, Anna Cohn Donnelly

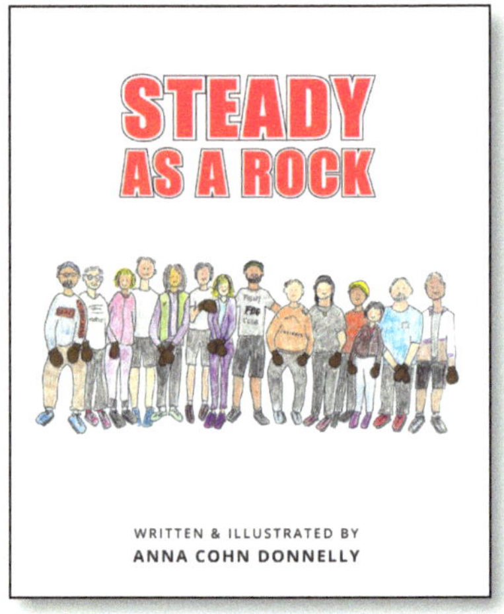

Steady as a Rock is a fully-illustrated inspiring story, told in the first person, of a group of senior citizens who find relief from the complications of Parkinson's and much more by regularly attending a boxing class entitled Rock Steady Boxing. By working out together, friendships abound and participants find they are no longer fighting alone the effects of the disease. The book documents the benefits of stepping out of your comfort zone.

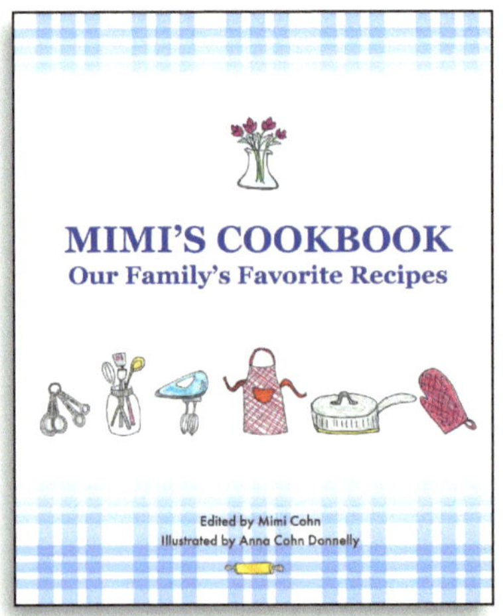

As she approached age 98, Mimi wanted to create something that would touch the whole family. Since we all love to eat and to cook, the idea of a cookbook that contained the family favorites made all the sense. **Mimi's Cookbook** is a collection of more than sixty odd favorites with illustrations.

Ozzie, a black mutt, tells his story of being adopted by the large and active Cohn family from Jack's Dog Farm and finding adventure and love in his new home, particularly with the youngest child Julie who arrived after he did. This is a heartwarming tale, filled with illustrations, of life on four paws.

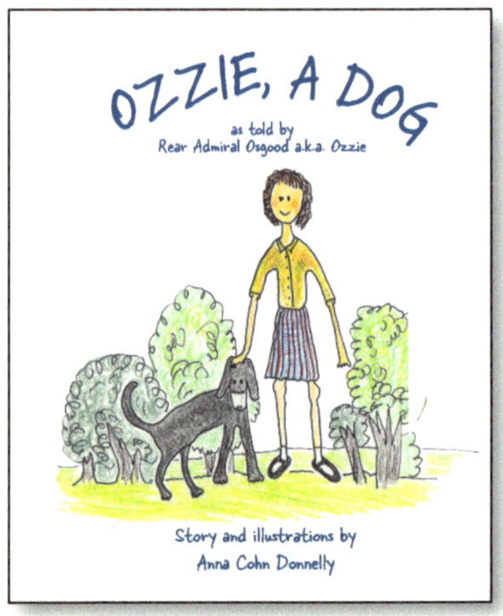

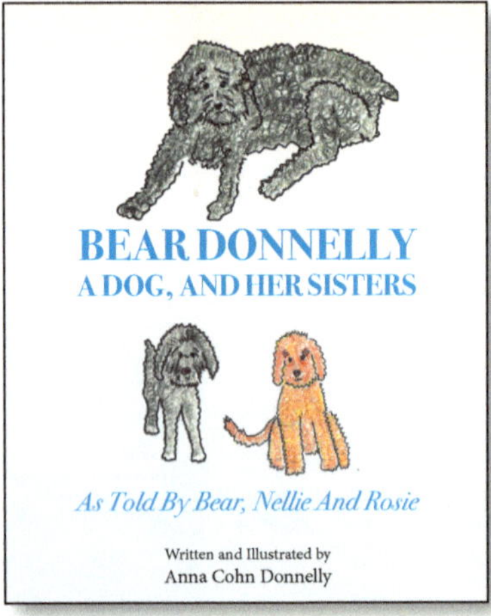

Bear Donnelly, A Dog, and Her Sisters, illustrated story told by Bear Donnelly, a 14 year old Bouvier de Flanders, of her life in the Donnelly household. Some of Bear's stories are happy ones, and some are not. Bear's younger sisters, Nellie and Rosie, also tell a bit about their lives.

Books by author & illustrator,
Anna Cohn Donnelly

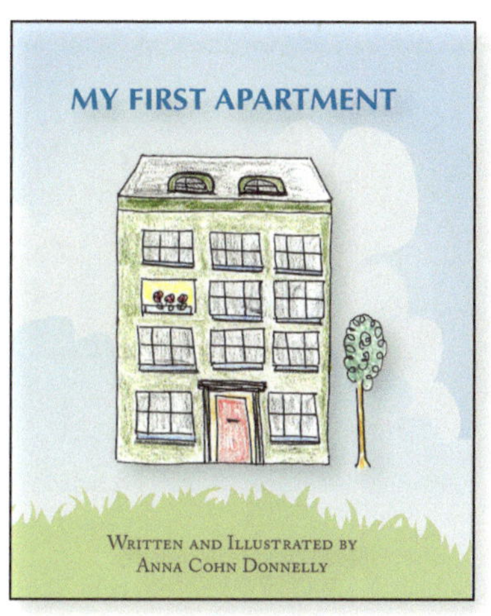

Having secured her first, real full time job, the youngest of four was leaving home to live downtown in an apartment with a school buddy. Rather than lecture her on the do's and do not's of living on her own, the author decided to cull advice from her older siblings and cousins and distill it in a short book. Written from the daughter's perspective, and fully-illustrated, *My First Apartment* offers guidance to those starting out on their own.

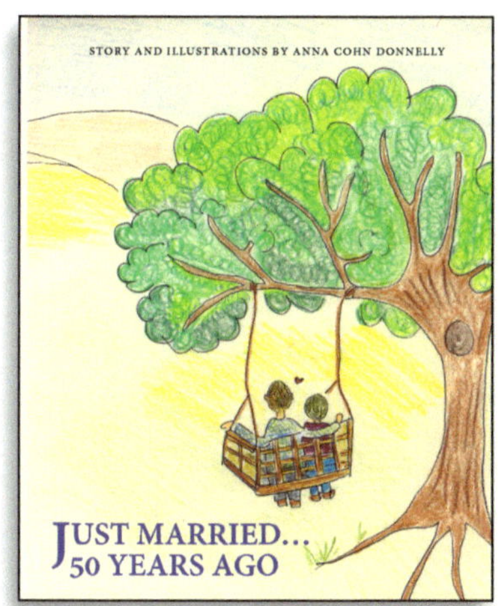

From the moment they met, David and Naida were in love. *Just Married…50 Years Ago*, a fully-illustrated book, follows them through their first fifty years and documents the best that a marriage and committed partnership can offer.

Amy was the fourth child of five, with two older brothers and an older sister and a younger one. She and her sister Anna, fourteen months her senior, had a profound impact on each other. *Our Sister Amy*, fully-illustrated, provides glimpses into the early years of their lives together and characterizes the best that sisters can offer each other as they grow up, even as they compete and strive for independence.

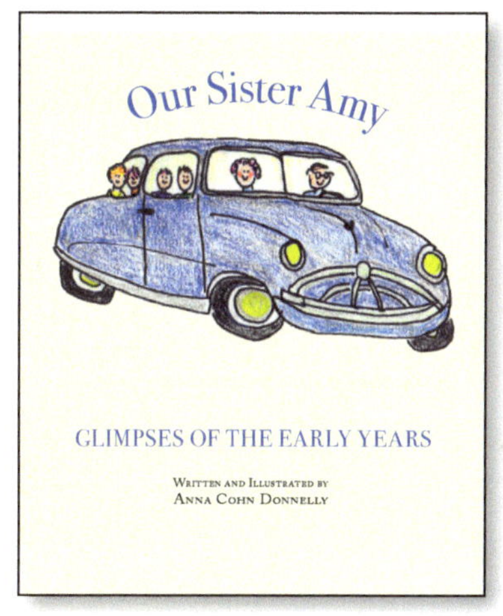